# *The* HEALTHY *BACK* BOOK

**Elizabeth Sharp** is a Chartered Physiotherapist with many years of practical experience. She has two thriving physiotherapy practices in London.

**Max Logan** is an internationally renowned photographer whose work has appeared in numerous publications.

# The *HEALTHY* *BACK* BOOK

## Simple Exercises for an Active, Pain-Free Back

**Elizabeth Sharp**

Grad. Dip. Phys., MCSP, SRP

Photographs by
**Max Logan**

ELEMENT

Shaftesbury, Dorset ● Rockport, Massachusetts
Brisbane, Queensland

© Elizabeth Sharp and Max Logan 1993

Published in Great Britain in 1993 by
Element Books Limited, Longmead, Shaftesbury, Dorset

Published in the USA in 1994 by Element, Inc.,
42 Broadway, Rockport, MA 01966

Published in Australia in 1994 by
Element Books Limited for Jacaranda Wiley Limited,
33 Park Road, Milton, Brisbane, 4064

Designed and typeset by Phil Payter Graphics
Printed and bound in Great Britain by the Bath Press
British Library Cataloguing in Publication data available
Library of Congress Cataloging in Publication data available

ISBN 1–85230–444–8

# *Contents*

# *Foreword*

*It gives me great pleasure to write the foreword for this most useful book which raises the whole question of health as opposed to disease. As a clinician I spend most of my time in diagnosing and treating disease. There is so much disease around that we tend to spend little time in thinking about prevention and healthy attitudes to living. It is of note that back pain for example is a very major cost of morbidity; 60 million working days are lost per annum due to back pain. This means that anything that can cut down this enormous financial burden should be viewed positively. In these days of starved resources and stringent cut backs we should all endeavour to support healthy attitudes of living.*

*Elizabeth Sharp has always had a very positive approach to health; in her treatment of patients she has emphasized prevention. Key words in her approach are exercise to keep fit, weight loss and attention to muscle tone. In this book she has endeavoured to produce strong arguments for a healthy approach to living. She has emphasized the need for regular exercise and the importance of this is clear for all. I support the programmes that are here described and hope that the readers will gain enormously from the knowledge that these chapters contain.*

**Dr Hedley Berry,** FRCP
Consultant Rheumatologist
96 Harley Street
London W1
Kings College Hospital
London SE5

# *Preface*

The idea for *The Healthy Back Book* evolved through many years of treating people with back pain and more recently, in the last four years, through running regular back classes for my patients once they had recovered sufficiently from the acute attack of back pain. Reaching a pain free state was only half way to full recovery as it was readily apparent that patients returned to the practice with recurrent attacks of back pain, often more frequently as the years went by. It was necessary to take people one step further along the path to recovery by teaching them how to strengthen their own back and stomach muscles in order to give vital stability to the spine and go some way to prevent future painful episodes. It was also an opportunity (at the right moment when the pain had gone but was fresh enough in the memory) to educate patients in preventative measures such as good posture, good lifestyle exercises, the correct weight for their height and some basic understanding of body mechanics and anatomy. I have found through experience that it takes about three episodes of back pain for a person to take themselves seriously in hand and accept that they must do something themselves to get fit with exercise and weight loss to keep themselves pain free.

Back pain continues to present challenges in diagnosis to the entire medical and paramedical professions. When is the pain due to a bulging disc? When is it due to blocked and inflamed facet joints and torn ligaments? When is it due to muscle spasm from bad posture and muscle imbalance? When is it due to 'wear and tear' type arthritis? These are some of the questions which have to be answered by orthopaedic surgeons, neurosurgeons, physical medicine specialists, GPs, physiotherapists, osteopaths and chiropractors who assess and treat patients who are 'back pain sufferers'. Because there are so many specialists in the field of back pain there are an equal number of treatments and 'cures' prescribed. Each individual has his or her own ideas and methods.

Twenty five years ago back pain was thought to be caused by sprained ligaments and sore muscles and the term 'lumbago' was used to describe low back pain. The treatment prescribed then was heat, massage and exercises. Sometimes the diagnosis was a 'slipped' disc and the patient was often immobilized in a corset or plaster of Paris jacket for several weeks. If that failed, surgery was performed to remove the disc and fuse the two adjacent vertebrae with a bone graft from the hip. Recovery was slow with several weeks spent flat in bed and then very cautious exercises. Thereafter strenuous activity was not recommended.

Today mechanical problems such as blocked joints are treated very successfully by different types of manual therapy. Rest is prescribed for short periods only, in the acute phase. It is vital to preserve mobility. Chartered physiotherapists have the advantage of a very broadly based training of which manipulation is a part and they work in close contact with their medical colleagues. I think that most physiotherapists who manipulate would agree that our method is based on the principle of the use of minimal force to achieve the desired result.

Back pain is often due to a combination of factors, such as blocked joints, weak muscles and muscle spasm. The patient will therefore require a combined treatment approach which could include some of the following techniques: manipulation, massage, muscular re-education, posture correction, electrotherapy, ice or heat, acupuncture, weight loss or a change in lifestyle. Each symptom is treated logically step by step with the most acute symptoms resolved first until full recovery is achieved.

Today most therapists would advocate non-invasive treatment whenever possible, with surgery being performed only as a last resort when there is evidence of nerve root damage.

Having taken my patients through to the final stage of recovery with back classes, I am certain from the comments they make that regular exercise helps to avoid recurrence of back trouble. They find to their surprise that the exercises are easy and quite fun to do even if they groan a bit at the beginning. They enjoy the company of others in the class and benefit from hearing about other people's problems and successes. If they do come back to me in later months or years with pain again it is often with the regret that they were fine while they were doing the exercises regularly but lapsed into trouble when something happened, like a new job or a move, which made them give up the routine of exercising. Gradually they became unfit, put on weight and the pain came back. I have myself had back trouble since I suffered a prolapsed disc as a physiotherapy student after a heavy fall skiing on ice. I can vouch for the fact that strong back exercises and stretching have kept me fit and working as a physiotherapist ever since. I have had three sons, run a marathon and actively partaken in sports such as swimming, tennis, windsurfing, waterskiing and snow skiing throughout my life. I believe that anyone can recover from back pain and attain an active life if they are prepared to devote ten minutes a day to following the advice given in this book.

# Acknowledgements

My indebtedness goes to my physiotherapy colleagues Lynnette France and Robyn Hill for their expert advice and help in the choice of exercises, running the back classes and reading the manuscripts; to my secretaries Karen Jones, Georgia Livesey and Jennifer Halvorsen for typing manuscripts; to Liz Capon for her support and advice on terminology; to Alan Glaser of Advance Seating for lending us the chair and desk used in the photographs; to Max Logan, without whose beautiful photographs and endless encouragement and advice this book would not have been written; and finally to my family for their backing and support and their help in editing the manuscripts.

# *Basic anatomy and biomechanics*

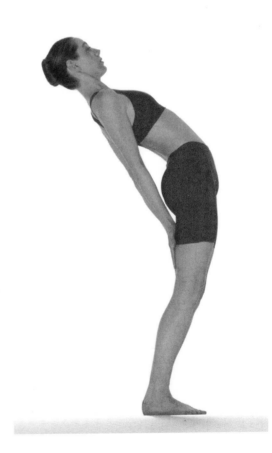

# Basic anatomy and biomechanics

*The spine*

## The Spine

The spinal column consists of seven cervical, twelve thoracic, five lumbar, five sacral and four coccygeal vertebrae, ranging from the base of the skull to the sacrum. Seen from the front, the normal spine is straight. Seen from the side, the spine is 'S' shaped. The neck curve is concave posteriorly as is the lumbar curve. The thoracic curve is convex posteriorly.

The spine is formed thus to withstand the considerable stress of loading. The lumbar vertebrae are the largest in the spinal column. This is because they carry all the weight of the body above the sacrum. They are strongest when maintained in the 'normal curve' and become weakened when flexed.

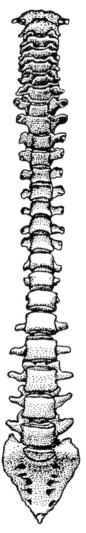 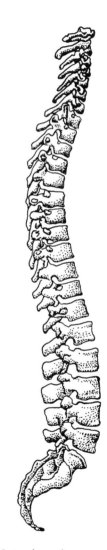

Spine anterior view        Spine lateral view

# Basic anatomy and biomechanics

*The lumbar vertebra*

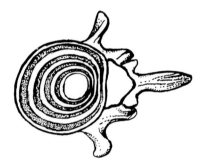

Cross section vertebra with disc

### The lumbar vertebra

The vertebra is constructed in such a way that it is as light as possible but with greatest density along the lines of force where weight is transmitted. A vertical section through the vertebral body would show many air spaces. The three spinous processes are for the attachment of muscle and ligament and, together with the vertebral body, form the roughly triangular shaped spinal canal enclosing the spinal cord.

# Basic anatomy and biomechanics

*The facet joints*

## The facet joints

Each vertebra locks into place with the next one through facet joints on either side. These joints have flat shearing surfaces which glide and slide on each other during movement of the spine. They can become blocked or damaged from incorrect loading and painful due to inflammation. Treatment such as expert spinal manipulation can help to clear blocked joints and reduce pain.

Persistent overloading through incorrect posture can cause wearing and an X-ray will show roughened articular surfaces and narrow spaces between the joints. These worn joints may be pain free most of the time and flare up only in a stressful episode. Further pain and degeneration may be avoided by adopting sensible postural habits and maintaining strong muscular support for the spine through regular exercise.

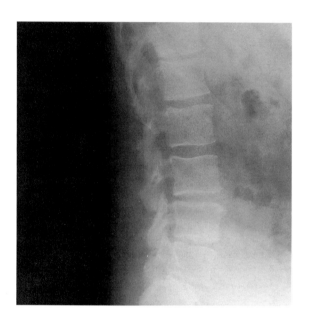

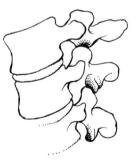

Facet joints interlocking

# Basic anatomy and biomechanics

*The disc*

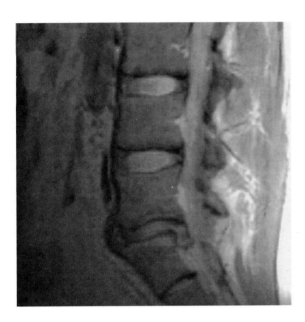

## The disc

The disc is sandwiched between each pair of vertebrae. It is a natural shock absorber and consists of a central gelatinous substance (the nucleus) surrounded by thick bands of fibrous tissue holding it in place under pressure. The nucleus can move in all directions depending on the position of the spine. If it bulges backwards towards the nerves and spinal cord (such as in forward bending or, worse still, forward with a twist), pressure may be exerted on the nerves, causing pain and damage.

Extreme pressure may cause the disc to squeeze out (herniate) permanently, causing nerve compression, requiring surgery to remedy the pain and resultant damage.

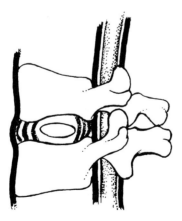

Ligaments and disc between two vertebrae

# Basic anatomy and biomechanics

## *The disc*

The disc is constantly loaded when the body is in the upright position and gravity exerts an inexorable downward force. This flattening force causes fluid to be lost from the disc with resultant narrowing. The young disc rehydrates while unloaded in the lying position. Thus we are all taller in the morning than we are at the end of the day. When older, the more permanent loss of disc height may lead to compression and wearing of the facet joints.

# Basic anatomy and biomechanics

*The nerves/The ligaments*

**1**

### The nerves

Branches of nerves come out from the spinal cord at each junction between the vertebrae.

Each branch is a power supply to a different section of skin, muscle, tendon and bone, transmitting sensation, muscular strength or pain.

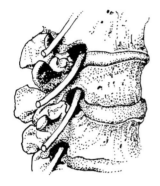

Lateral view foramen and nerve root

### The ligaments

The ligaments are tough bands of fibrous tissue that bind one vertebra to another. In the spine there are two long columns running from the base of the skull to the sacrum along the anterior and posterior surfaces of the vertebrae. There are also smaller ligaments bridging each adjacent posterior process. They afford the ultimate linking of the vertebral column. They are very strong, but not normally elastic.

# Basic anatomy and biomechanics

*The muscles*

## The muscles

The extensor muscles support the spine against gravity and hold the body in the upright position. They are attached to the back of the vertebrae and spinous processes in layers from the base of the skull to the sacrum. The very deep muscles are short and connect adjacent vertebrae; the superficial muscles are long columns which run on either side of the vertebral column to give the distinctive contour of the back.

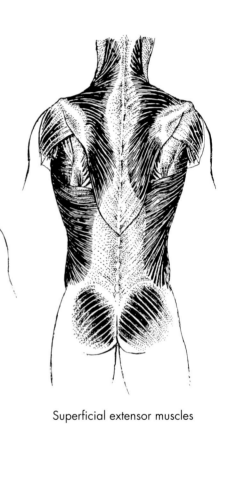

Superficial extensor muscles

Deep extensor muscles

CHAPTER 1

# Basic anatomy and biomechanics

## *The muscles*

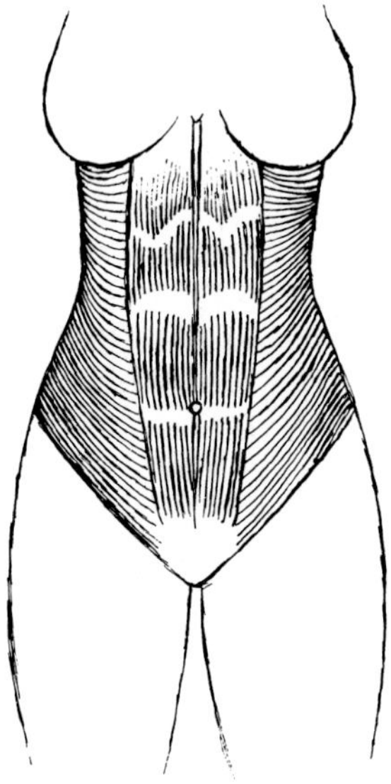

Abdominal muscles

The abdominal (stomach) muscles support the spine by regulating pressure within the abdomen, especially in actions such as pushing, lifting, coughing or sneezing. There are layers of oblique sheets of muscle which function like a girdle and activate rotation, and thick vertical bands attaching from the ribs to the pelvic rim which work to flex the body.

Weak stomach muscles are frequent contributors to back trouble. They become flabby and lazy with weight increase.

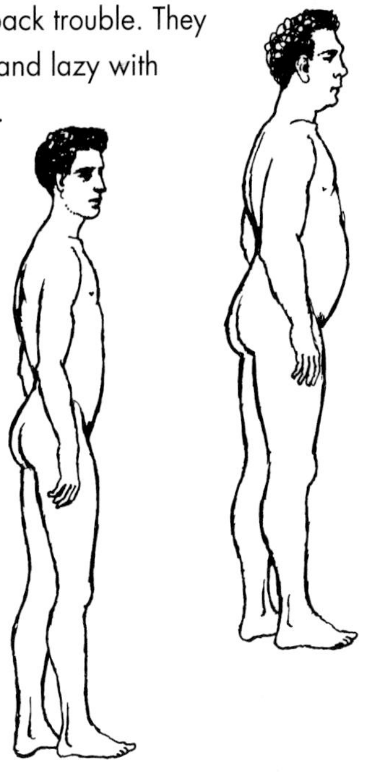

# Basic anatomy and biomechanics

*Functional movement*

## Functional movement

The range of functional movement of the spine is determined by the cumulative effect of the movement of the individual vertebrae. Mobility is also determined by joint, muscle and ligament flexibility. Flexibility can be improved and maintained by regular exercise and stretching.

Dysfunction results from adaptation to chronic pain.

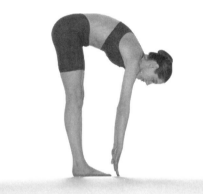

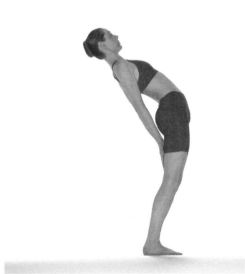

# Basic anatomy and biomechanics

*Functional movement*

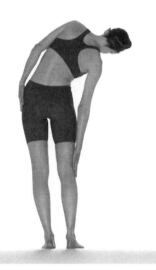

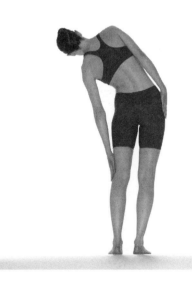

# Basic anatomy and biomechanics

*Loading*

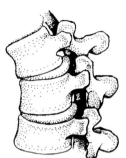

## Loading

The best way to damage your spinal joints or discs is to bend from the waist, keeping your knees straight and twisting to pick up something heavy.

**In this position it is possible to transmit 1000kg or more through your lower lumbar joints and discs depending on the strength or weakness of your stomach muscles.**

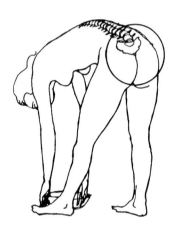

Long term sitting also causes major loading problems as greater pressure is passing through the lower lumbar vertebrae in sitting than in standing.

**100 per cent upper body weight passes through lumbar vertebrae 4 and 5 in standing, 140 per cent in good sitting and 190 per cent in bad sitting.**

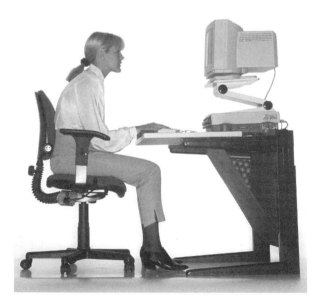

# *The exercises – introduction*

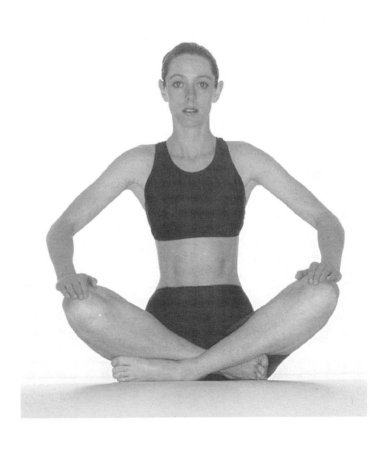

# The exercises – introduction

*Why do exercises?*

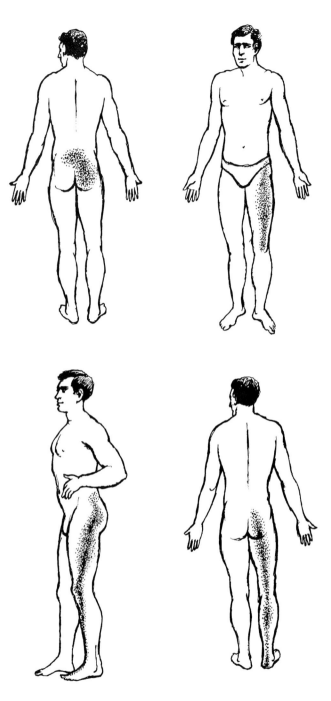

'Mapping' the pain on a body chart

## Why do exercises?

The spine is a strong working component of the body needing muscular strength and stability to support the joints and prevent damage. Almost certainly back and stomach muscles will weaken after a period of pain and rest from normal activity. As these are the muscles that support the spine they will therefore need to be strengthened. Pain should be relieved by exercise if it is due to stiff or blocked facet joints and it should clear fairly quickly, in a few days, unless there is excessive inflammation or degeneration. A painful facet joint may cause the spine to shift sideways to avoid loading. This can be seen on examination and may need manipulation to clear if the exercises alone do not work. Seek advice from your physiotherapist or doctor.

Even the pain from a bulging disc can be relieved if pressure is removed by exercising the joint in the correct way to free the trapped nerve, but it may take weeks rather than days to resolve. It is possible to determine where the trouble is coming from by 'mapping' the pain

# The exercises – introduction

*Why do exercises?*

on a body chart. Only the grossly prolapsed disc will resist pain relief from exercise, when surgery may be necessary. X-rays and MRI (magnetic resonance imaging) scans, which identify the problem, are very useful to confirm the diagnosis

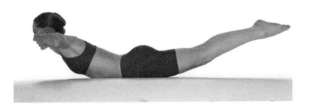

**The back muscles** hold the spine upright in the erect position and constantly work against gravity. They only become seriously weakened after a period of prolonged bedrest. Following spinal surgery it is most important to strengthen the back muscles to take strain away from the spinal ligaments, which will have been cut during surgery, to enable them to heal slowly over a period of months.

# The exercises – introduction

*Why do exercises?*

**The abdominal muscles** support the spine by regulating the pressure inside the abdomen and supporting the internal organs. They work to about 50 per cent capacity until really needed and we are lazy about using them. It is therefore very easy for the stomach muscles to be slack and much weaker than you realize, and they will remain so unless you regularly strengthen them. If they are weak they let you down during activities such as coughing, sneezing, lifting and pushing, and the pressure inside the abdominal cavity rises, causing compression of the lumbar discs. This problem becomes much worse if you put on weight, have abdominal surgery or you fail to strengthen the muscles after having a baby.

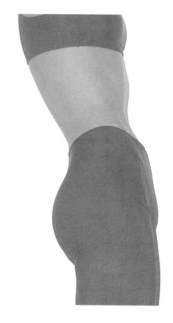

# The exercises – introduction

*How to do the exercises*

## How to do the exercises

Even if you are in a painful episode try to do the gentle warm-up easy exercises (Chapter 3). They will stop you from seizing up by keeping the joints lubricated and the blood circulating. Take plenty of short rests lying down but exercise for about five minutes every hour. Change position often, alternating between walking and lying. Sit only if supported with a small cushion in the small of the back, and avoid bending. The more pain you have, the more you should do the exercises 'little and often'. Your pain should begin to subside with the pain focus centralized to the back and out of the leg. Then you may add the very gentle strengthening exercises. If this routine does not ease your pain you must seek advice from your physiotherapist or doctor.

**Intermediate exercises** When your pain has settled, so that it is only intermittent and mild, you should be able to progress to the more difficult exercises, which begin to seriously strengthen muscle (Chapter 4). You may be back at work but you will still need to

# The exercises – introduction

*How to do the exercises*

exercise often. It may still be necessary to lie down on the office floor for ten minutes from time to time to rest the back. Continue the intermediate exercises at home once a day for three to four weeks to consolidate your recovery.

**The ten minute maintenance routine**
When you are almost or completely pain free move on to the strong and fast maintenance routine (Chapter 5) that you should do daily for six months and maybe for ever. This routine should become part of your daily life, like brushing your teeth, until you feel unhappy if you forget it. Ten minutes of hard exercise a day is a small price to pay for a pain free back. You should also be able to get back to all normal activities and sport, but remember to start carefully.

# The exercises – introduction

*How to do the exercises*

**The office exercises** (Chapter 7) are good to do at any time after you get back to work. Sitting is the worst position for the spine and the best way to relieve pressure is to move and exercise regularly. Try to do the sitting exercises every hour and get up and move around frequently. If you have a sedentary job, spending 80 – 100 per cent of your working day sitting, it is vital to have a good working chair which supports the lumbar spine, on a forward tilting seat, to avoid wear and tear. When choosing your chair look for adjustable seat height and angle, adjustable backrest height and angle, five feet with casters, a swivel seat and armrests if you write or use a keyboard.

# The exercises – introduction

*The stretches*

## Why do stretches?

Stretches are necessary to restore full flexibility to the joints of the spine and hips and to ensure that joint surfaces and articular cartilage remain healthy by being compressed from one end of the range to the other. If this normal rolling compression is not maintained through movement the cartilage lining becomes worn and thin resulting in 'crunchy' sounds inside the joint. This is the first step in the degenerative process of 'wear and tear'. As we use, on average, only 60 per cent of the available range of movement it is most important to stretch after an episode of back pain, which will further reduce that range. Stretches should only be started when the acute pain is mild or settled. They are not popular, as a stretch done correctly feels uncomfortable.

# The exercises – introduction

*The stretches*

### How to stretch

Stretching should always be done cautiously and slowly, stopping at the point where the stretch pain is felt and holding for twenty seconds or more. If you hold for a shorter period of time the desired effect will be limited. Stretch daily and never bounce at the end of the stretch or you may cause damage to the muscle tendon.

# *Easy exercises for a painful back*

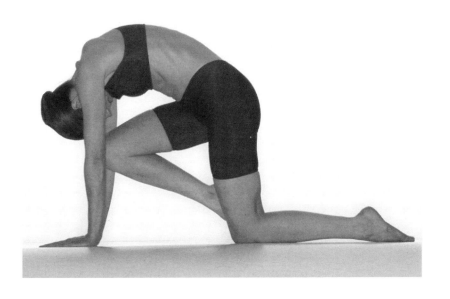

# CHAPTER 3

# Warm-up

*Knee Hugging*

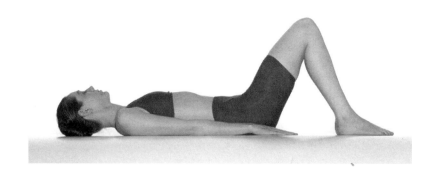

Lie on your back with your knees bent.

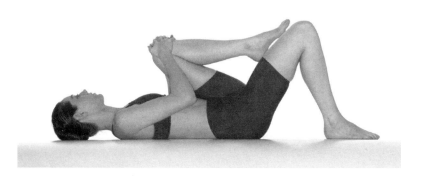

Take your left knee in both hands and hug it up towards your chest. Repeat ten times.

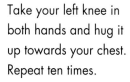

# Warm-up

*Knee Hugging*

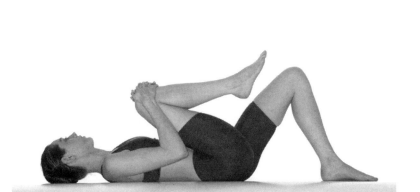

Lower the left leg and hug your right leg in the same way. Repeat ten times.

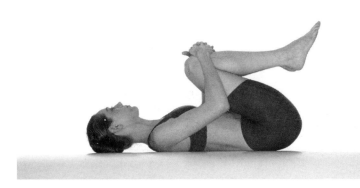

Now hug both knees together towards your chest. Repeat ten times.

# Warm-up

*Knee rolling*

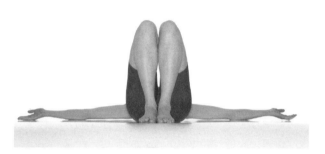

Lie on your back with your knees bent and your arms out to the sides. Keep your shoulders flat on the floor and your feet and knees together.

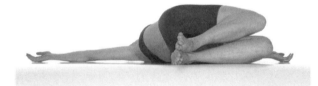

Roll your knees to the right as far as you can and touch the floor if possible.

Now roll your knees back to the left to touch the floor if possible.

Keep your shoulders flat but allow your hip to lift so that you rotate the spine. Roll right to left in a smooth rhythmic movement ten times.

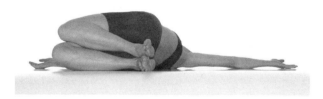

# Warm-up

*Pelvic rocking in lying*

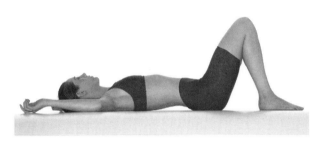

Lie on your back with your knees bent and your hands beside your head.

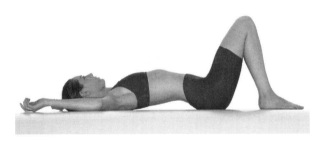

Arch your back to make a hollow under your waist keeping your shoulders flat and your bottom down.

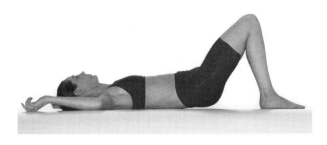

Now push down to flatten your back against the floor while tightening your stomach muscles.

Repeat ten times.

# Warm-up

*Pelvic rocking in kneeling*

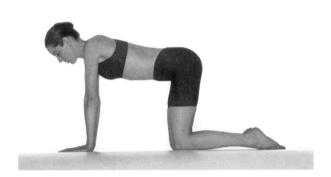

Kneel on all fours with your weight evenly distributed between your hands and knees.

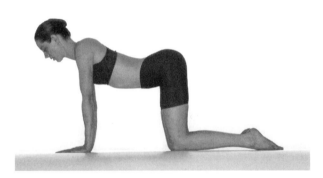

Keeping your elbows locked, make a hollow in your lower back.

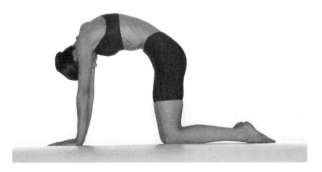

Now arch up your back, trying to localize the movement to your lower back. Rock up and down rhythmically. Repeat ten times.

CHAPTER

3

EASY EXERCISES FOR A PAINFUL BACK ———————— 28

# Warm-up

*Passive extensions*

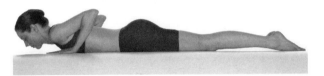

Lie face down on the floor with your hands under your shoulders, in the 'press-ups' position, and your elbows bent.

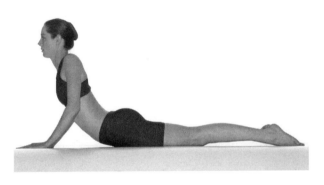

Keeping your hips as flat as possible, push down on your hands and straighten your elbows to arch your back. Push up as high as you can. Repeat ten times.

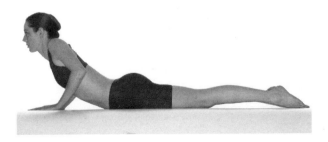

You may only be able to reach as high as this at first.

# Stomach muscle strengthening exercises

*Static stomach tightening*

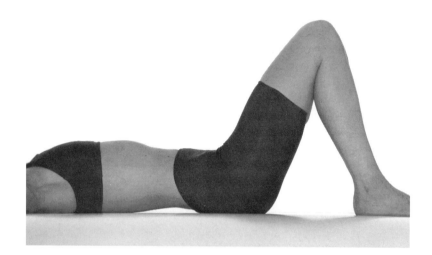

Lie on your back with your knees bent.

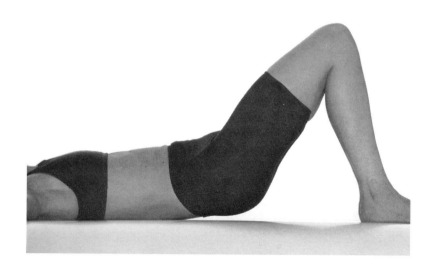

Press your back down firmly on to the floor and tighten your stomach muscles as hard as you can.

Count out loud to ten while you breathe normally.

Repeat the exercise ten times.

# Back muscle strengthening exercises

*Back extension in kneeling*

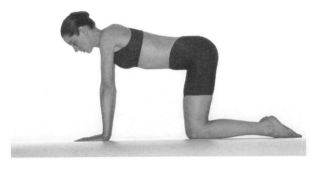

Kneel on all fours on the floor with your weight evenly distributed between hands and knees. Keep your knees and hands apart.

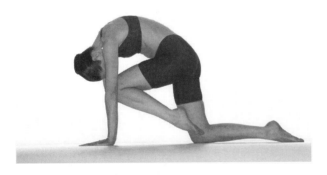

Bend your left knee up towards your chin as high as you can.

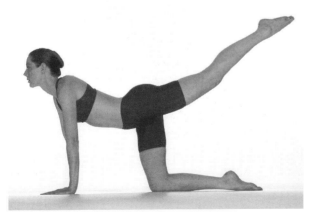

Now stretch your left leg backwards, straightening your knee and arching your back. Do not twist your hips.

# Back muscle strengthening exercises

*Back extension in kneeling*

Bring your left knee back to the floor.

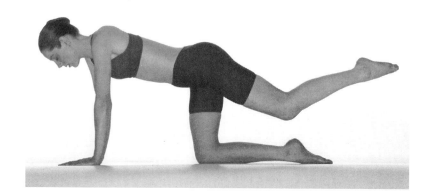

Start again from the beginning.

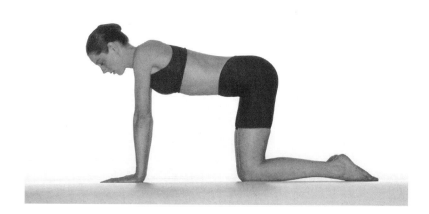

# Back muscle strengthening exercises

*Back extension in kneeling*

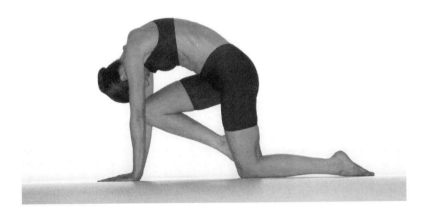

Bend your right knee
up towards your chin
as high as you can.

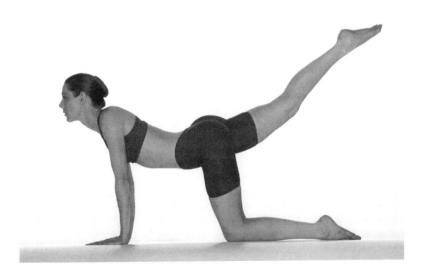

Stretch your leg
backwards keeping
your knee straight and
arching your back.
Bend and stretch
each leg ten times
alternately.

33

# *Exercises for a recovering back*

CHAPTER 4

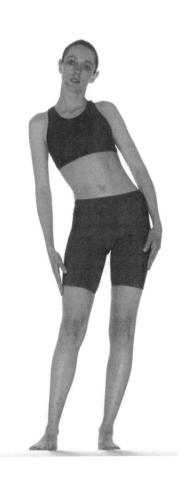

35

# Warm-up

*Knee hugging*

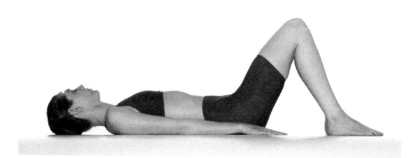

Lie on your back with your knees bent.

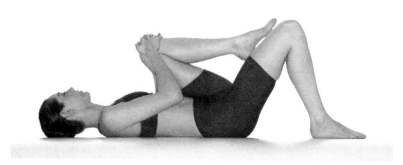

Take your left knee in both hands and hug it up towards your chest. Repeat ten times.

# Warm-up

*Knee hugging*

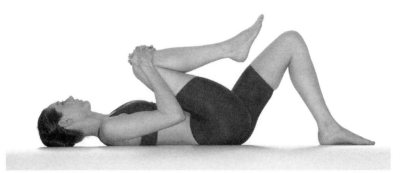

Lower the left leg and hug your right leg in the same way. Repeat ten times.

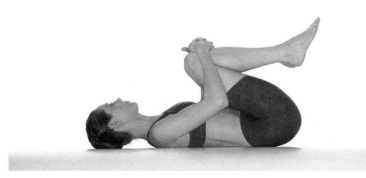

Now hug both knees together towards your chest. Repeat ten times.

# Warm-up

*Knee rolling*

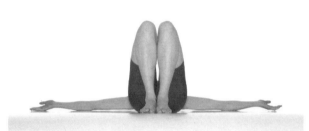

Lie on your back with your knees bent and your arms out to the sides. Keep your shoulders flat on the floor and your feet and knees together.

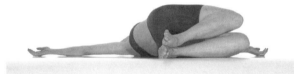

Roll your knees to the left as far as you can and touch the floor if possible.

Now roll your knees back to the right to touch the floor if possible.

Keep your shoulders flat but allow your hip to lift so that you rotate the spine. Roll right to left in a smooth rhythmic movement ten times.

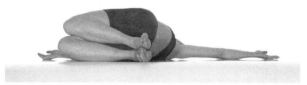

# Warm-up

*Pelvic rocking in lying*

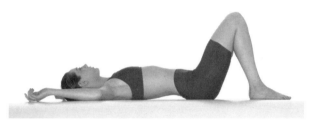

Lie on your back with your knees bent and your hands beside your head.

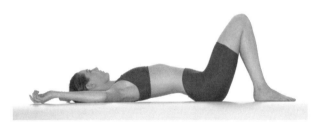

Arch your back to make a hollow under your waist keeping your shoulders flat and your bottom down.

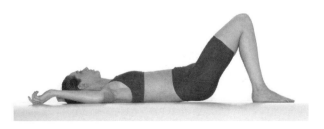

Now push down to flatten your back against the floor while tightening your stomach muscles.

Repeat ten times.

# Warm-up

*Pelvic rocking in sitting*

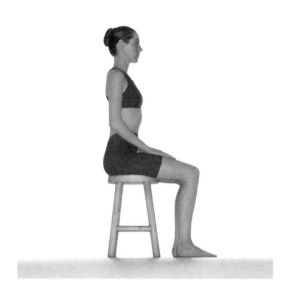

Sit on a firm chair or stool. Arch your back making a hollow at your waist.

Now slump and curl your lower back as much as possible.

Repeat arching and slumping in a rocking movement ten times.

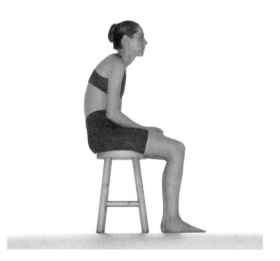

# Warm-up

*Side bends*

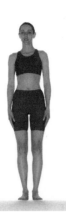

Stand with your feet slightly apart and your weight evenly balanced between both feet.

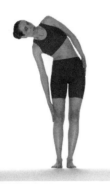

Slide your right hand down your leg until your fingers reach the knee crease. Keep your heels on the floor and do not twist your body.

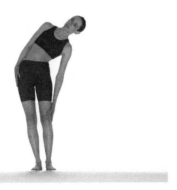

Come back to the upright position and slide your left hand down the left leg until your fingers reach the knee crease.

Repeat this movement smoothly and slowly from right to left ten times.

# Warm-up

*Side shunts*

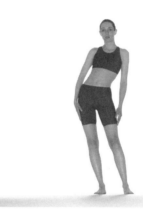

Stand with your feet about 18 inches apart and your weight evenly balanced between both feet.

Keeping your shoulders level and your arms relaxed, shunt your right hip out to the side.

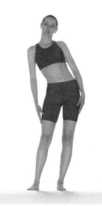

Return to the midline and shunt your left hip out to the side.

Repeat side shunts smoothly, right to left, ten times.

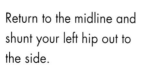

## Warm-up

*Backward rotations*

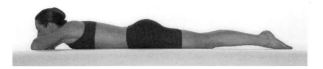

Lie face down with your hands under your chin.

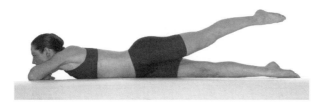

Lift your left leg backwards, keeping the knee straight.

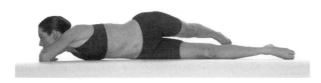

With your shoulders as flat as possible, cross your left leg over the right leg until you can touch the floor with your toe.

*Backward rotations*

Lower the left leg back to the floor.

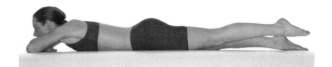

Now lift the right leg backwards, keeping the knee straight.

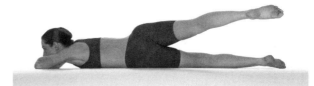

Keeping your shoulders flat, cross your right leg over your left leg until your foot touches the floor.

Repeat this movement with alternate legs ten times.

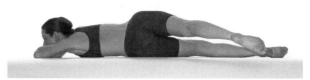

# Warm-up

*Passive extensions*

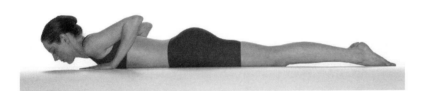

Lie face down on the floor with your hands under your shoulders, in the 'press-ups' position, and your elbows bent.

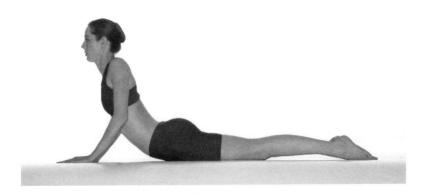

Keeping your hips as flat as possible, push down on your hands and straighten your elbows to arch your back. Push up as high as you can. Repeat ten times.

# Warm-up

*Sitting rotations*

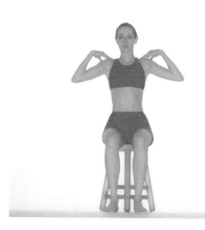

Sit on a firm chair or stool with your fingers resting on your shoulders. Keep your feet firmly on the floor and your knees pointing forward.

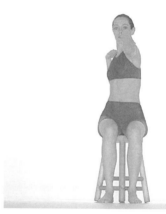

Rotate your shoulders to the right as far as you can without turning your head.

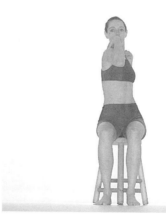

Now turn and rotate your shoulders as far to the left as you can while keeping your head still. Rotate right and left in a swinging movement ten times.

# Stomach strengthening exercises

*Static stomach tightening*

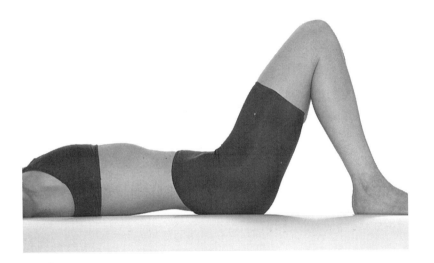

Lie on your back with your knees bent.

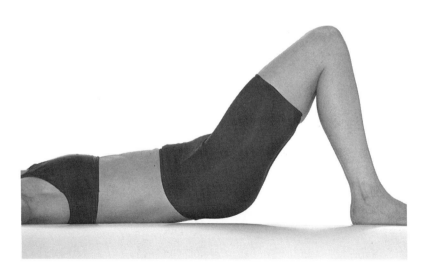

Press your back down firmly onto the floor and tighten your stomach muscles as hard as you can.

Count out loud to ten while you breathe normally.

Repeat the exercise ten times.

# Stomach strengthening exercises

*Three position stomach crunches*

Lie on your back with your knees bent and your feet off the floor with one foot crossed over the other. Take both hands up towards your knees.

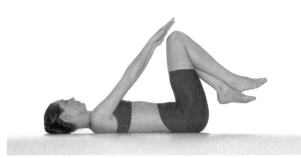

Lift and curl your head and shoulders, taking your hands over the top of your knees. Hold for five seconds, keeping stomach muscles very tight.

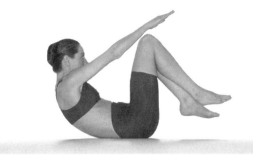

Go back to the start position in between each curl.

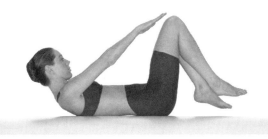

# Stomach strengthening exercises

*Three position stomach crunches*

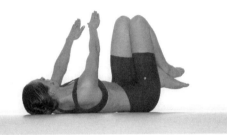

Now take both hands towards the outside of the left knee.

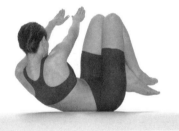

Lift up and curl head and shoulders, taking both hands over the outside of your left knee. Hold for five seconds, keeping stomach muscles tight.

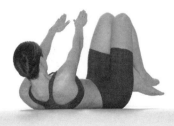

Lower and rest for a second.

# Stomach strengthening exercises

*Three position stomach crunches*

Now take both hands towards the outside of the right knee.

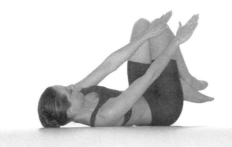

Lift up and curl head and shoulders, taking both hands over the outside of your right knee. Hold for five seconds, keeping your stomach muscles tight.

These three positions make a **set**. Repeat each set three times with as little rest in between each movement as possible.

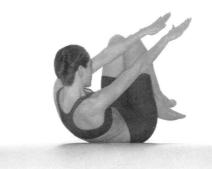

# Stomach strengthening exercises

*Knees to chest stomach crunch*

**This exercise needs to be done slowly with lots of control and starting with a small range of movement. If your back arches off the floor you are not tightening your stomach muscles hard enough.**

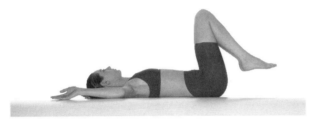

Lie on your back with your knees bent and feet off the floor. Keep your hands on the floor above your head.

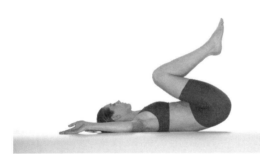

Lift both your knees up on to your chest as high as you can so that your bottom lifts off the floor slightly.

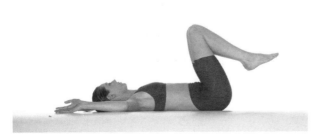

Keeping your back flat on the floor and your stomach muscles working hard, lower your knees to the midline position. Raise and lower your knees in this small arc of movement ten times.

# Back strengthening exercises

*Back extensions in kneeling*

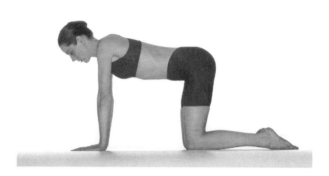

Kneel on all fours on the floor with your weight evenly distributed between hands and knees. Keep your knees and hands apart.

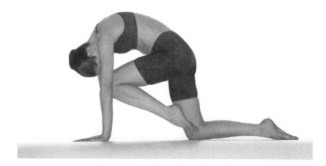

Bend your left knee up towards your chin as far as you can.

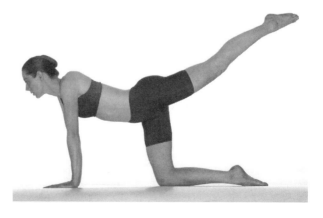

Now stretch your left leg backwards, straightening your knee and arching your back. Do not twist your hips.

# Back strengthening exercises

*Back extensions in kneeling*

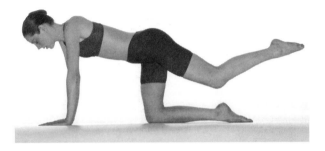

Bring your left knee back to the floor.

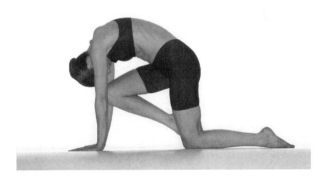

Do the same movement with your right knee. Try to take your knee as near to your chin as possible.

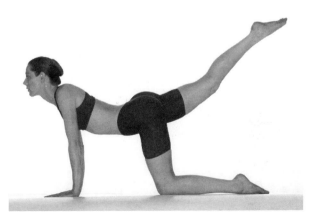

Now stretch your right leg backwards keeping your knee straight and arching your back. Bend and stretch each leg alternately ten times.

# Back strengthening exercises

*Single leg extensions*

Lie face down with
your hands under your
chin.

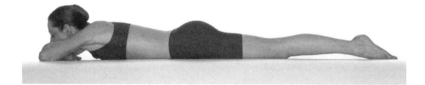

Keeping your knee
straight and both your
hips on the floor, lift
your left leg up as high
as you can.

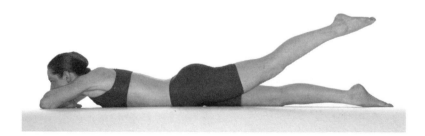

# Back strengthening exercises

*Single leg extensions*

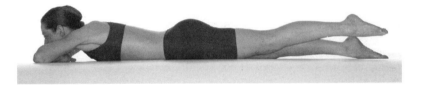

Lower the left leg to the floor. Repeat the lifts 5–10 times, increasing as you feel stronger.

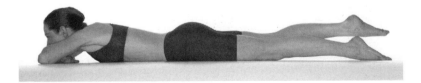

Now lift the right leg.

# Back strengthening exercises

*Single leg extensions*

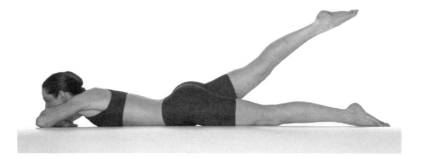

Lift as high as you can without twisting your hips.

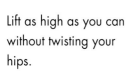

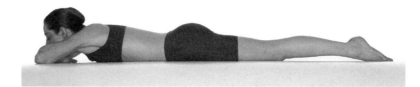

Lower the right leg and repeat the lifts 5–10 times, increasing as you feel stronger.

# Back strengthening exercises

*Head and shoulder lifts*

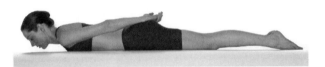

Lie face down with your
hands clasped behind your
back.

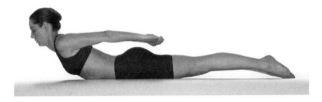

Lift your head and shoulders
while stretching your arms
backwards. Your eyes should
be looking down so that you
do not strain your neck.

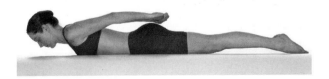

Lower slowly and repeat the
exercise, without rest, ten
times.

# Stretches

*Hamstring stretch*

**The hamstring muscle lies at the back of the thigh.**

Lie on your back and clasp firmly with both hands behind your right knee. Keep your head relaxed on the floor.

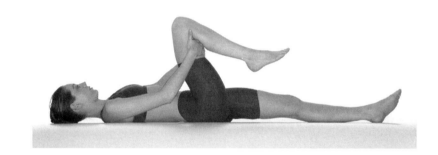

Straighten your right leg by contracting your knee muscle (quadriceps) tightly. Hold for twenty seconds.

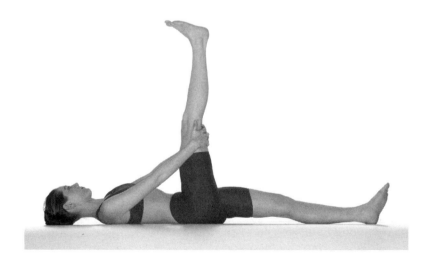

## Stretches

*Hamstring stretch*

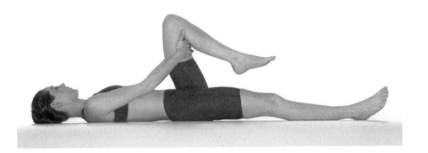

Now stretch your left
leg in the same way.

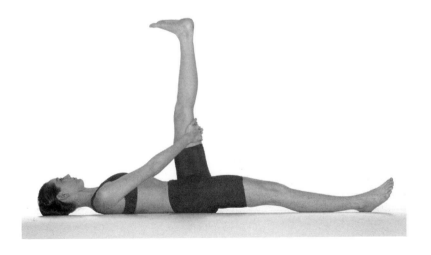

Lock your knee as
straight as possible by
tightening your thigh
muscle. Keep your
head and right leg
relaxed on the floor.
Hold for twenty
seconds.

# Stretches

*Quadriceps stretch*

**The quadriceps muscle is at the front of the thigh.**

Lie face down and clasp your left foot in both hands.

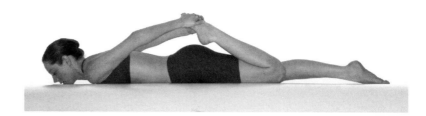

Pull your heel in towards your buttock, lifting your knee slightly. Hold for twenty seconds.

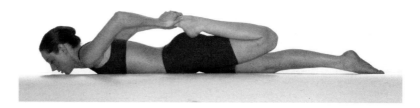

## Stretches

*Quadriceps stretch*

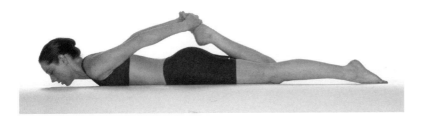

Repeat the same exercise with the right foot in both hands.

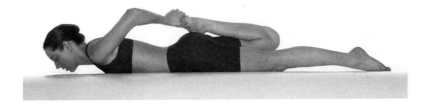

Pull your heel firmly in towards your buttock, lifting the knee slightly. Hold for twenty seconds.

# Stretches

*Yoga stretch*

**This position will stretch several lower back and hip muscles.**

Sit on the floor with your left leg straight and your right knee bent with your right foot placed outside your left knee. Twist your body to the **right**, positioning your left elbow against your right knee and stretching your right hand out to the side while rotating your shoulders to the **right** as far as possible. Hold for twenty seconds.

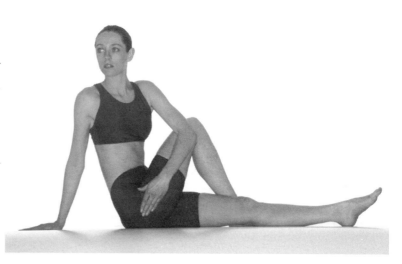

Now stretch to the opposite side. Straighten your right leg and bend your left knee, placing your left foot on the outside of your right knee. Twist your body to the **left**, placing the right elbow against the left knee and stretching your left arm out to the side while rotating your shoulders to the **left** as far as possible. Hold for twenty seconds.

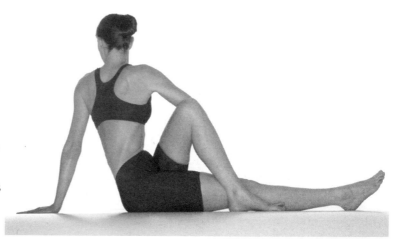

# Stretches

*Hurdle sitting*

**This position stretches lateral back, hip and thigh muscles.**

Sit on the floor with your right leg rotated outwards and your left leg rotated inwards with your knee pulled back as far as you can in the hurdle position. Try to have your left thigh in line with your shoulders. Pull yourself as upright as possible with your left hand on your left knee. Hold for twenty seconds.

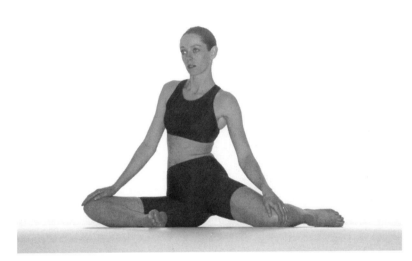

Stretch to the opposite side with left leg rotated outwards, right leg rotated inwards with your knee pulled back as far as possible in the hurdle position. Pull yourself as upright as possible with your right hand on your right knee. Hold for twenty seconds.

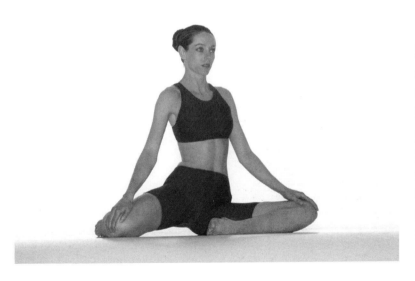

# Stretches

*Crossed leg sitting*

**This stretch is for
the muscles on
the inside of the
thighs.**

Sit on the floor with
your feet crossed
and your hands resting
on your knees.

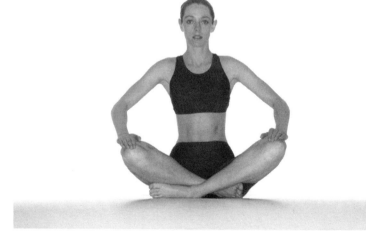

Push your knees down
towards the floor with
pressure from your
hands. Hold for twenty
seconds.

# Stretches

*Straight leg rotations*

**This is a good stretch for the lower back, particularly when there is persistent one-sided pain and stiffness. It will also stretch stomach, hip and thigh muscles.**

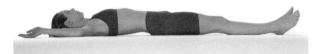

Lie on your back with legs straight and your hands resting above your head.

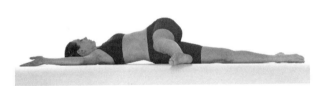

Keeping your shoulders flat on the floor, lift and rotate your left leg across your right leg keeping it straight and touching the floor with your foot. Hold for twenty seconds.

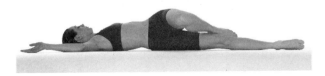

Bring your left leg back to the floor.

# Stretches

*Straight leg rotations*

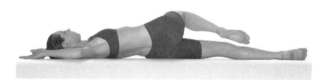

Begin the stretch to the opposite side.

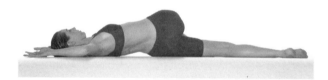

Keeping your shoulders as flat as possible, lift and rotate the right leg across the left, keeping it straight and touching the floor with your foot. Hold for twenty seconds.

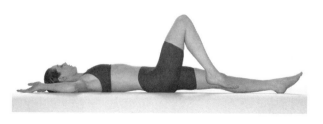

Bring your right leg back to the floor.

# *The ten minute maintenance routine*

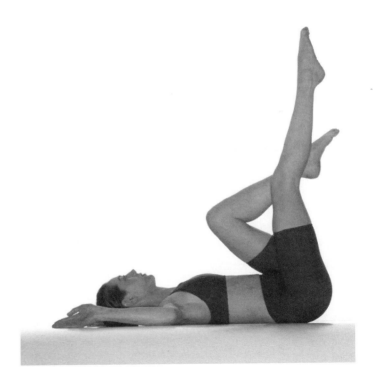

# The ten minute maintenance routine

- Double knee hugging × 20                                     20 seconds
- Knee rolling × 20                                            20 seconds
- Half press-ups × 10                                          20 seconds
- Full back extension with hands on ears × 20                 30 seconds
- Three position stomach crunches with hands on ears × 5       2 minutes
- Knees to chest stomach crunch × 20                          30 seconds
- Reverse stomach crunches                                      1 minute
- Vertical cycling                                              1 minute
- Hamstring stretch                                             1 minute
- Quadriceps stretch                                            1 minute
- Yoga stretch                                                  1 minute
- Slump stretch                                                 1 minute

                                               10 minutes

These exercises need to be done fast and without rests to fit into the ten minute slot but with some practice this can be achieved. The exercises which follow should be used as a guideline to build up the most appropriate maintenance routine to suit the individual. The selection above does fulfil the necessary criteria of warm-up, back strengthening, stomach strengthening and stretching exercises, but there may be some other exercises in previous chapters which suit your needs better. The best answer is to adapt the list to suit yourself.

# Warm-up

*Knee hugging*

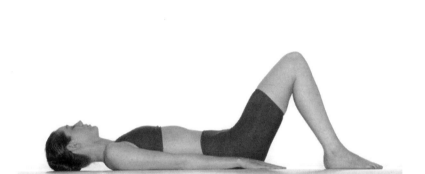

Lie on your back with your knees bent.

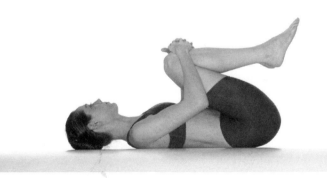

Hug both knees up to your chest. Repeat twenty times with no rest.

# Warm-up

*Knee rolling*

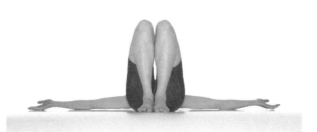

Lie on your back with your knees bent and your arms out to the sides. Keep your shoulders flat on the floor and your feet and knees together.

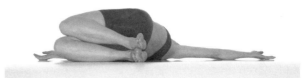

Roll your knees to the right as far as you can and touch the floor if possible.

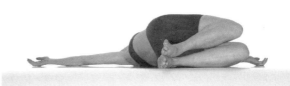

Now roll your knees back to the left to touch the floor. Keep your shoulders flat but allow your hip to lift so that you rotate your spine.

Roll right to left rhythmically twenty times.

# Warm-up

*Passive extensions*

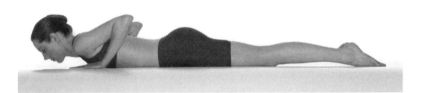

Lie face down on the floor with your hands under your shoulders (in the 'press-ups' position) and your elbows bent.

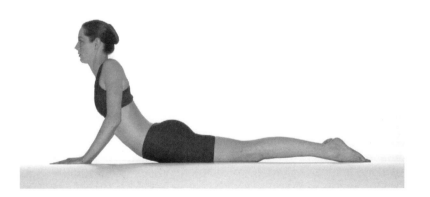

Keeping your hips as flat as possible, push down on your hands and straighten your elbows to arch your back. Push up as high as you can. Repeat ten times.

71

# Back muscle strengthening exercises

*Full back extension with hands on ears*

Lie face down with your legs straight and your hands on your ears.

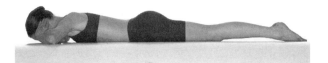

Lift your head and shoulders and both legs together, making an arch with your whole back. Keep your eyes looking down so that you do not strain your neck.

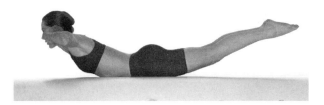

Lower for a second and lift again. Repeat the lifts, without resting, twenty times.

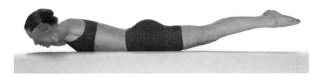

# Stomach strengthening exercises

*Stomach crunches with hands beside ears*

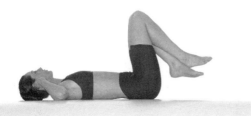

Lie on your back with your knees bent.
Lift your feet slightly off the floor and cross one foot over the other. Put your hands beside your ears.

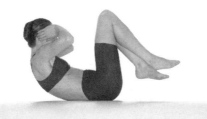

Lift up and curl your head and shoulders, keeping your neck as relaxed as possible. Hold for five seconds.

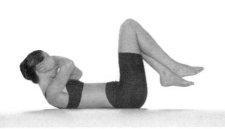

Lower briefly.

# Stomach strengthening exercises

*Stomach crunches with hands behind ears*

Now lift and rotate your body to the right, taking your elbows towards your right knee. Hold for five seconds, tightening your stomach muscles hard.

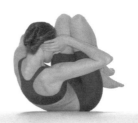

Lower again briefly.

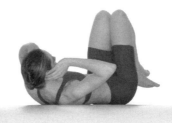

Now lift and rotate your body to the left, taking your elbows towards your left knee. Hold for five seconds, tightening your stomach muscles hard.

These three positions form a **set**. Repeat each set five times.

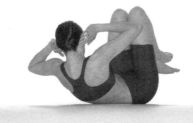

# Stomach strengthening exercises

*Knees to chest stomach crunches*

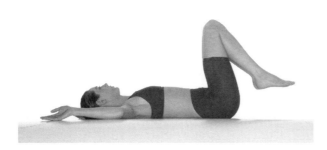

Lie on your back with your knees bent and feet off the floor. Keep your hands above your head.

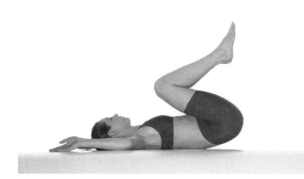

Lift both your knees up to your chest as high as you can so that your bottom lifts off the floor slightly.

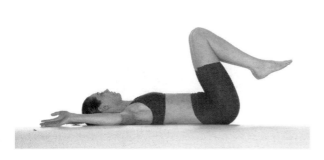

Keeping your back flat on the floor and your stomach muscles working hard, lower your knees slowly to the midline position. Raise and lower your knees smoothly in this small arc of movement twenty times.

# Stomach strengthening exercises

*Reverse stomach crunches*

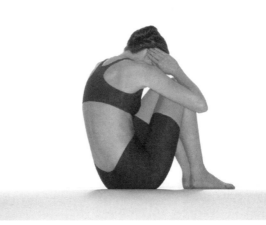

Sit on the floor with your knees bent and your heels tucked back as far as possible. Put your hands beside your ears and your chin on to your chest.

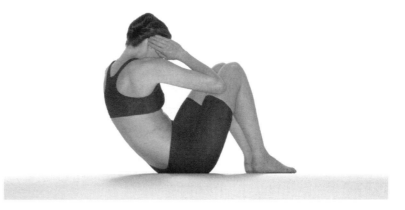

Keeping yourself in this tucked position, lower backwards slowly until you feel your feet wanting to lift. Stop immediately and hold for ten seconds.

# Stomach strengthening exercises

*Reverse stomach crunches*

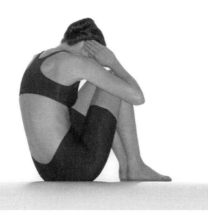

Come back up to sitting but remain in the tucked position.

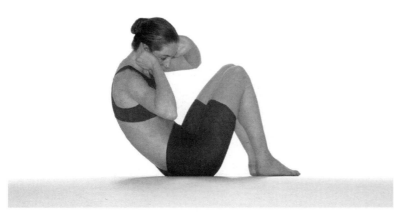

Now curl backwards but twist your body towards the right, keeping your feet on the floor. Hold for ten seconds.

# Stomach strengthening exercises

*Reverse stomach crunches*

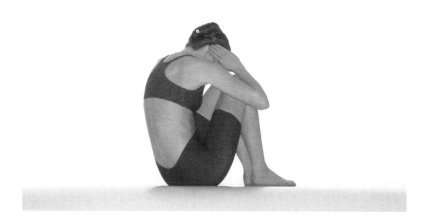

Come back up to sitting.

Now curl backwards in the tucked position but twist your body towards the left and keep your feet on the floor. Hold for ten seconds.

These three positions form a **set**. Repeat each set three times.

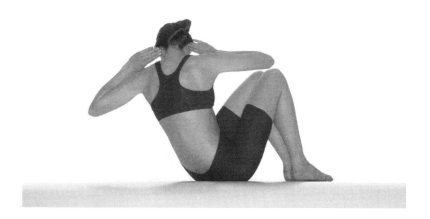

# Stomach strengthening exercises

*Vertical cycling*

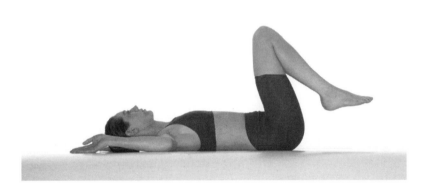

Lie on your back with your knees bent and feet off the floor.

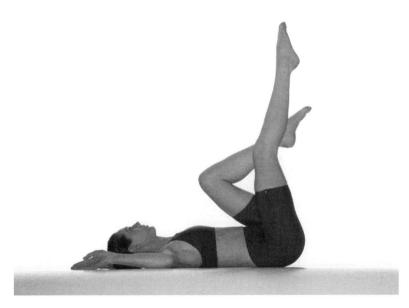

Stretch both legs up vertically but keep your knees bent.

# Stomach strengthening exercises

*Vertical cycling*

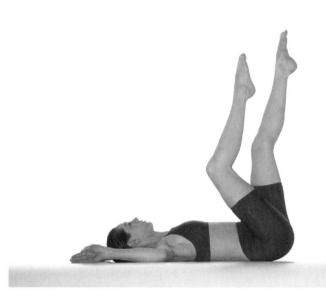

Start small cycling movements with your feet, keeping your legs vertical and holding your stomach muscles tight.

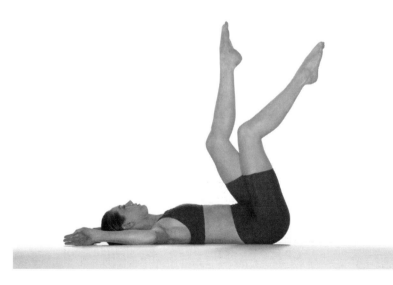

Cycle for thirty seconds non-stop. Do not allow your legs to go below the vertical line.

# Stretches

*Hamstring stretch*

**The hamstring muscle lies at the back of the thigh.**

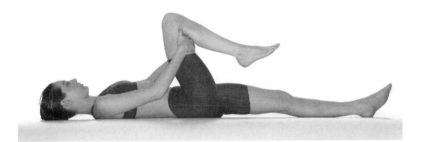

Lie on your back and clasp firmly with both hands behind your right knee. Keep your head relaxed on the floor.

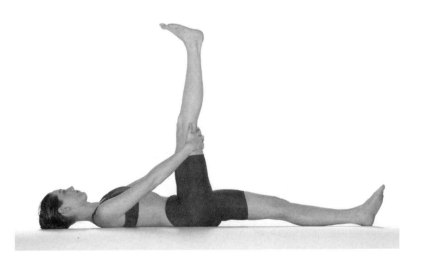

Straighten your right leg by contracting your knee muscle (quadriceps) tightly. Hold for twenty seconds.

81

# Stretches

*Hamstring stretch*

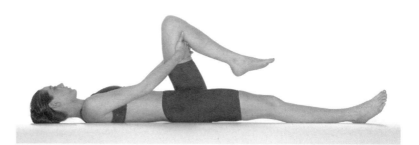

Now stretch your left leg in the same way.

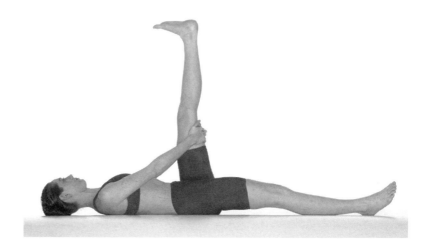

Lock your knee as straight as possible by tightening your thigh muscle. Keep your head and right leg relaxed on the floor. Hold for twenty seconds.

# Stretches

*Quadriceps stretch*

The quadriceps muscle is at the front of the thigh.

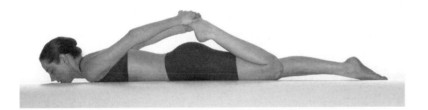

Lie face down and clasp your left foot in both hands.

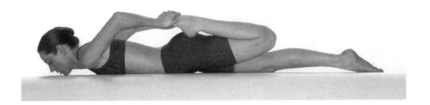

Pull your heel in towards your buttock, lifting your knee slightly. Hold for twenty seconds.

# Stretches

*Quadriceps stretch*

Repeat the same exercise with the right foot in both hands.

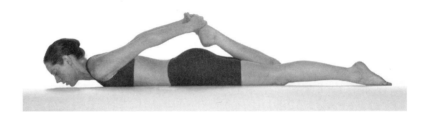

Pull your heel firmly in towards your buttock, lifting the knee slightly. Hold for twenty seconds.

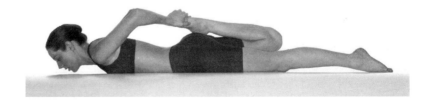

# Stretches

*Yoga stretch*

**This position will stretch several lower back and hip muscles.**

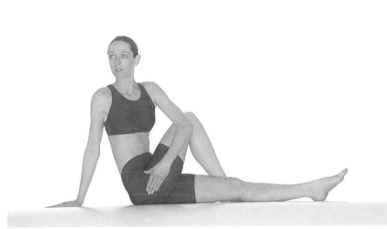

Sit on the floor with your left leg straight and your right knee bent with your right foot placed outside your left knee. Twist your body to the **right**, positioning your left elbow against your right knee and stretching your right hand out to the side while rotating your shoulders to the right as far as possible. Hold for twenty seconds.

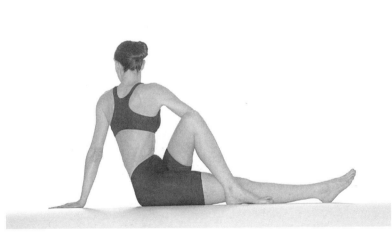

Now stretch to the opposite side. Straighten your right leg and bend your left knee, placing your left foot on the outside of your right knee. Twist your body to the **left**, placing the right elbow against the left knee and stretching your left arm out to the side while rotating your shoulders to the **left** as far as possible. Hold for twenty seconds.

# Stretches

*Slump stretch*

**This stretch must be done slowly and with caution. Do it in stages: first your chin down, then your knee straight and finally pull your foot up. You will feel a stretching sensation all the way from your buttock to your foot.
If it should cause real pain, stop.**

Sit on a firm stool or chair with your hands clasped behind your back and your chin tucked down on to your chest. Slowly straighten your right knee and pull your foot up. Hold for twenty seconds.

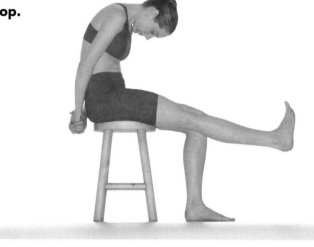

Now stretch the left leg. Remember to go into the stretch slowly and to hold for twenty seconds.

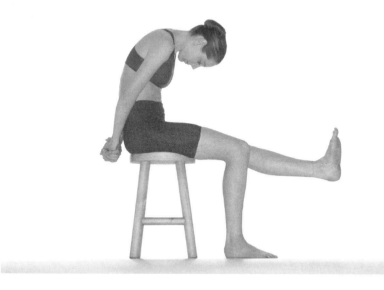

# *Mobility checks*

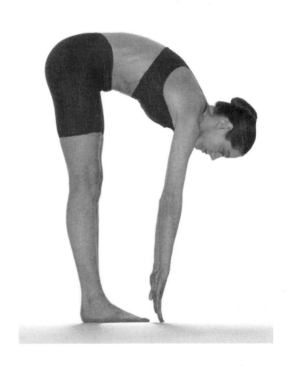

# Mobility checks

We all stiffen up as we get older. This is most likely due to the fact that on average we use only 60 per cent of the available range of body movement. When we are young we dash about playing sport, dancing, stretching and reaching and using every muscle and joint to the fullest range. As we get older our expectations change and our bodies become less mobile. This need not be the case if we stay healthy, take exercise and stretch on a regular basis. We all know people in their eighties who remain flexible through activity. They are the ones who look young and feel good.

**Use it or lose it.**

Once upon a time we could all do this....

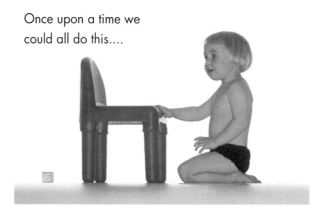

and this....

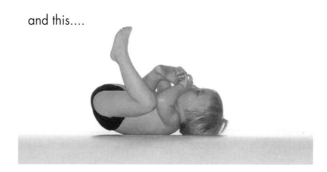

and this.

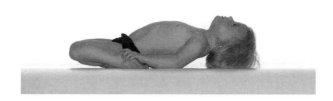

# Mobility checks

The following mobility checks are useful to do on a regular basis to gauge your general level of flexibility. Just do one of each, stretching as far as you can without causing pain and holding the position for only a short time. If anything feels stiff or hurts, try doing the stretches in **Chapter 4**.

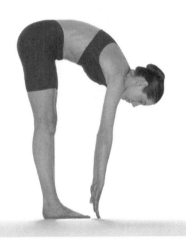

Stand with your feet slightly apart and slowly bend forwards to touch your toes, keeping your knees straight. Stop when you feel tightness.

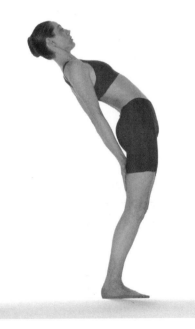

Bend backwards, sliding your hands down the backs of your legs and keeping your knees straight.

# Mobility checks

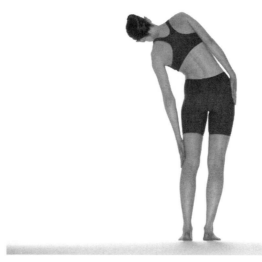

Bend sideways to the left, sliding your hand down the outside of your leg until it reaches the knee.

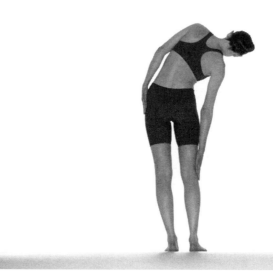

Bend sideways to the right, sliding your hand down the outside of your leg until it reaches the knee.

# Mobility checks

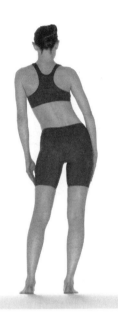

Stand with your feet apart and shoulders level and shunt your hip out to the right.

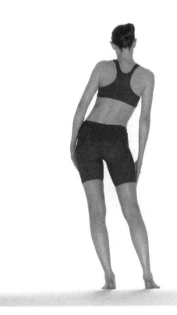

Stand with your feet apart and shoulders level and shunt your hip out to the left.

# Mobility checks

Sit on a firm chair or stool with your hands on your shoulders and twist your body to the right.

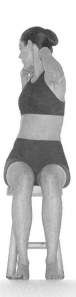

Now twist your body to the left.

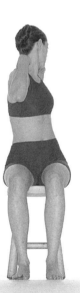

## Mobility checks

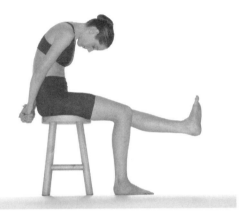

Sit on a firm chair or stool with your hands behind your back and your chin tucked down. Straighten your left knee and pull your foot up.

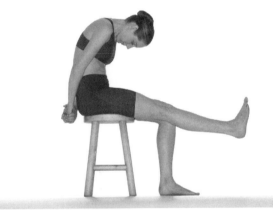

Now straighten the right knee and pull your foot up.

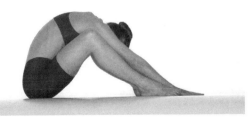

Sit on the floor with your knees bent and feet apart. Stretch your hands down to touch your toes, bringing your head between your knees.

# *Office exercises*

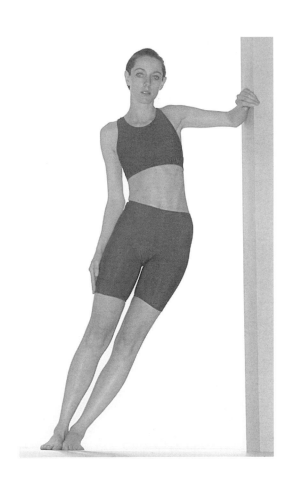

# Office exercises

*1. Sitting rotations*

If you have a job that involves a lot of sitting the following exercises can easily be done at your desk or on a chair in the office. They should be done hourly to prevent stiffness and pain building up. They can also be done at other times where long term sitting is necessary, such as in a plane or bus, or in your car if you stop at a convenient place on a long journey.

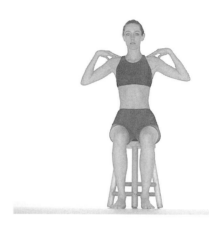

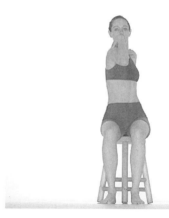

Sit on your office chair or a firm seat with your hands on your shoulders. Twist your body all the way round to the left and then all the way to the right in a swinging motion. Keep your head facing forward so that you do not strain your neck. Swing from left to right twenty times.

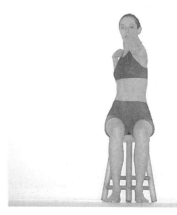

# Office exercises

*2. Rotation stretches*

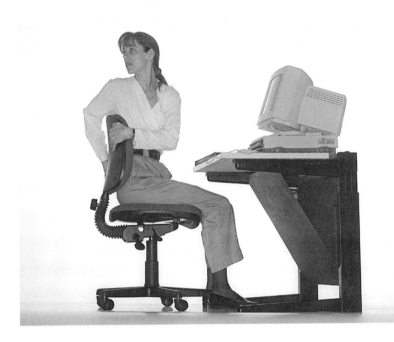

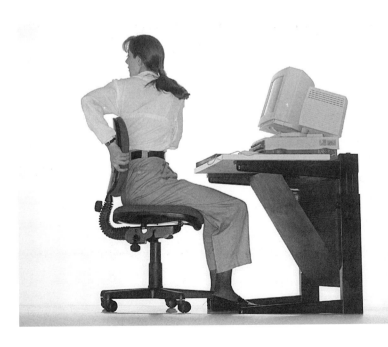

Sit on a firm chair with a back. Your office chair will be ideal. Start by sitting squarely on the seat. Now twist your upper body to the right, locking yourself around the back of the chair with both arms. Hold for twenty seconds. Then twist your body to the left and hold for twenty seconds. Turn as far as you can in both directions.

# Office exercises

*3. Side shunts in sitting*

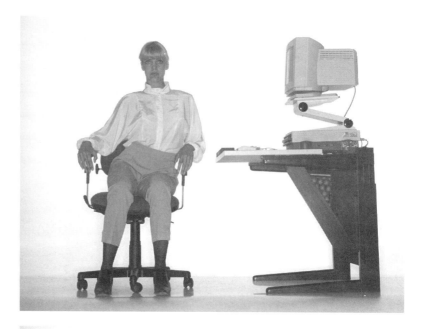

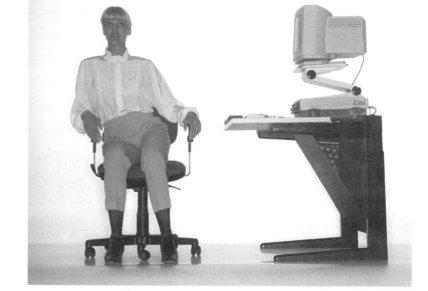

Sit on your office chair
and tilt all your weight
on to your left buttock
and then shift all the
weight over to the right
buttock. Keep your
shoulders level. Rock
right to left twenty
times.

# Office exercises

*4. Knee hugging in sitting*

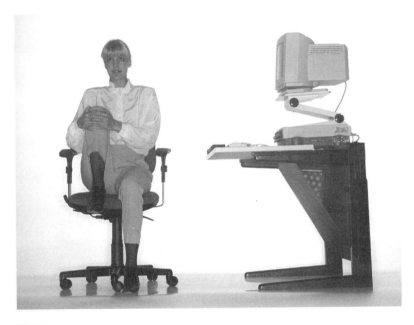

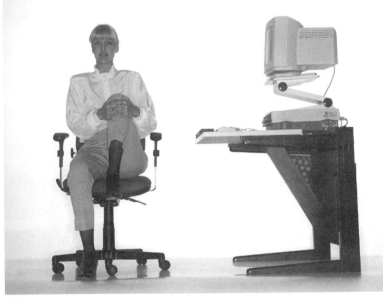

Sit on your office chair. Take your right knee in both hands and hug it up towards your chest ten times and then hug your left knee up towards your chest ten times.

# Office exercises

*5. Toe touching in sitting*

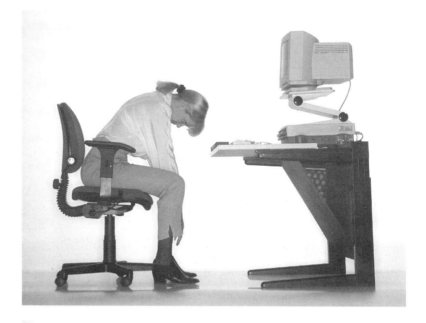

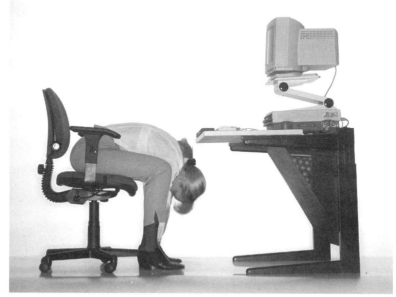

Sit on your office chair
and reach down to
touch the floor
between your feet.
Bend up and down ten
times.

# Office exercises

*6. Wall support shunts*

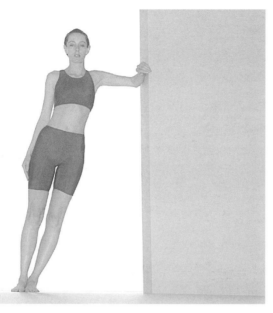

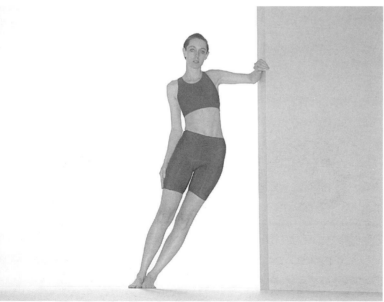

Stand next to the wall with your feet together and your left elbow supported on the wall. Your body should be at a slant, with your feet as a pivot. Shunt your left hip in towards the wall without twisting your body and then back to the midline again, repeating the exercise ten times. Now turn around and place your right elbow on the wall and repeat the exercise, shunting to the right ten times.

101

# Office exercises

*7. Pelvic rocking in sitting*

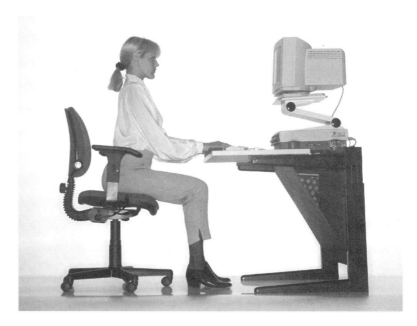

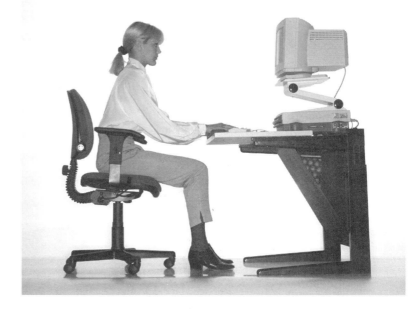

Sit on your chair and hollow your back as much as you can and then slump and flatten your back. Rock back and forwards, curling and arching your back ten times.

# Office exercises

## 8. Stomach tightening in standing

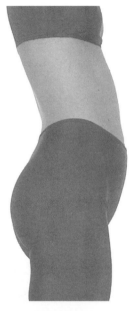

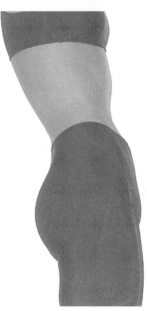

This exercise has been shown with the stomach exposed so that you can see the effect of the muscles tightening. The exercise can, of course, be done fully clothed and also in sitting and lying. The first position shows the stomach slack and protruding even in a slim person. To tighten the stomach try to flatten your back and pull the front of the stomach wall inwards. Hold tight for twenty seconds while counting out loud.

It is good to practise this while you are on the phone and you should eventually be able to hold it without effort for longer and longer periods. The back often aches when you have to stand for long periods but you will feel less back pain if you hold your stomach muscles in tight.

# *Good resting positions*

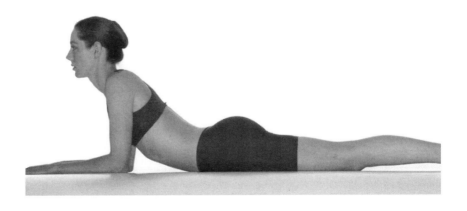

# Good resting positions

If your back is still intermittently uncomfortable or tires easily, the following resting positions should help to ease the pain and relax muscle spasm. Muscle spasm is very tiring. A timely ten minute rest may mean that you are able to stay working comfortably for a normal day. Stop and rest as soon as you feel pain building up and try to rest anyway two or three times within the working day until you feel fully back to normal. You can lie on the floor if necessary.

## Lying with pillows under the knees

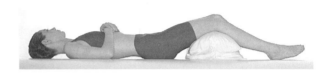

## Lying with legs on a chair

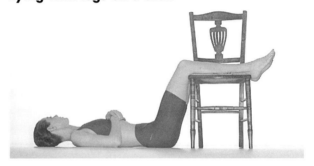

Lie on the floor with your hands on the floor in front of your shoulders. Prop yourself up onto your forearms so that your back is arched. This position will help to ease referred leg pain and centralize it to the back by decompressing the disc and removing pressure from the pinched nerve roots. It is also a useful position in which to read, play with the children or watch television. After practice, you should be able to maintain this position for several minutes.

## Prone resting position

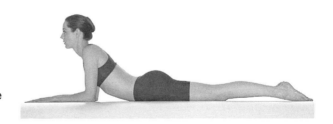

# *Posture*

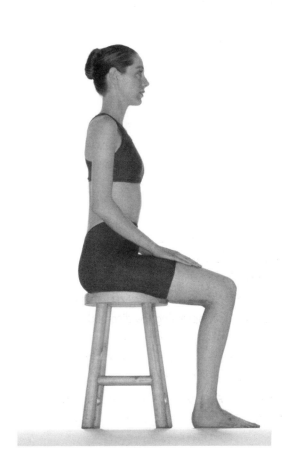

# Posture

If you value your back, make a habit of adopting good postural habits.

**1**. Sit like this...                    But not like this...

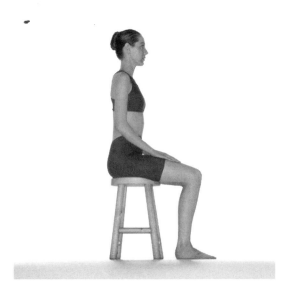        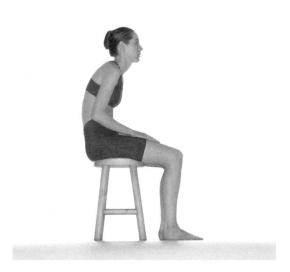

**2**. Lie like this...                    But not like this...

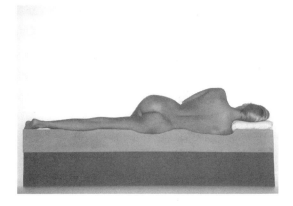        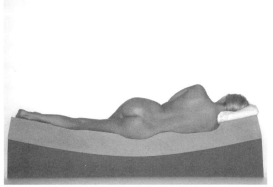

# Posture

**3.** Lift like this... But not like this...

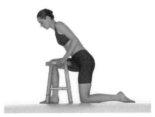 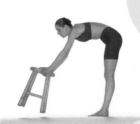

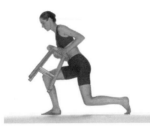 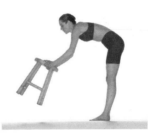

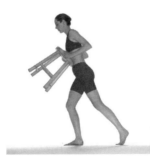 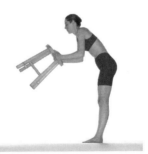

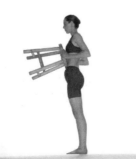 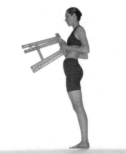

**4.** Sit at your desk like this...    But not like this...

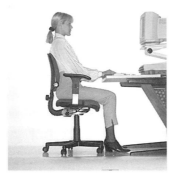 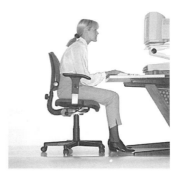

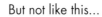

**5.** Sit in your car like this...    But not like this...

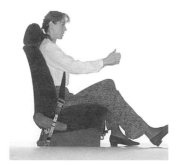 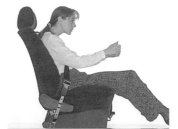

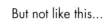

**6.** Lift and hold your baby like this...    But not like this...

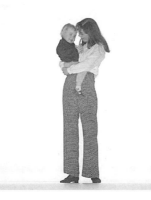 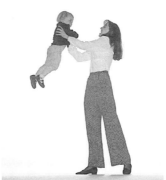

# Posture

**7.** Carry shopping like this...

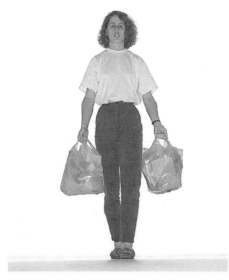

But not like this...

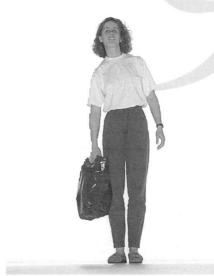

or like this

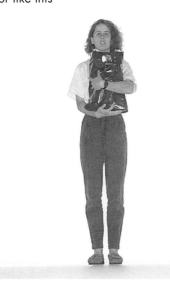

and not like this...

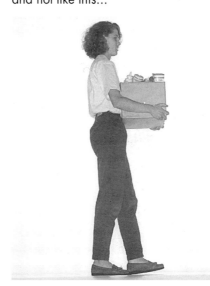

**8.** Always pick up
shopping like this

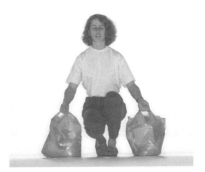

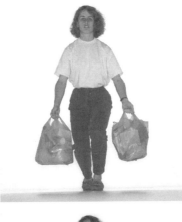

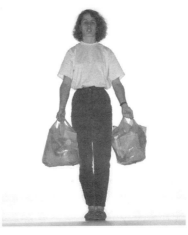